DR. JEFF KEYSAR, DC

# The Owner's Manual for Your Neck And Back

*How To Maintain A Healthy Neck & Back by Sitting, Sleeping, Exercising, and Working Properly, and What To Do If You Don't*

First edition

This book was professionally typeset on Reedsy.
Find out more at reedsy.com

# Contents

# Disclaimer

The information provided in this book is designed to provide helpful information on the subjects discussed. This book is not meant to be used, nor should it be used, to diagnose or treat any medical condition. For diagnosis or treatment of any medical problem, consult your own physician. The publisher and author are not responsible for any specific conditions that may require medical supervision and are not liable for any damages or negative consequences from any treatment, action, application or preparation, to any person reading or following the information in this book.

# I

# Instructions For Use (of Your Neck And Back)

# 1

# Introduction

Over the past twenty years in chiropractic practice, I've been asked the same questions by literally thousands of back pain patients. Questions like:

**Should I be using ice or heat?**

**What is the best mattress?**

**Are there any stretches I can do to help my back?**

**What's the best pillow to use?**

**Should I be taking any medicine for my back?**

**When can I exercise again?**

........and dozens more like these.

Why it took so many years I'll never know, but the day finally came when it dawned on me that having all of this information in one place to help back pain sufferers feel better, faster might be a good idea. And since I'm a practical person who appreciates "getting down to business," I figured writing in the style of an instruction manual would save everyone a lot of time, especially someone in pain who needs to feel better now, not tomorrow.

Inside these pages, you'll learn how to avoid the various forces that work on you throughout the day, making your back worse, and how to fix them so that pain and degeneration are minimized.

You'll learn why spinal bones don't necessarily go "out", but instead, you'll understand how joints get "stuck". You'll learn why exercises are often necessary to truly make your back healthy, but not the typical exercises you'd do in a gym setting.

You'll learn how your pillow, bed, car seat, work chair, shoes, vehicle, daily tasks, and even your hobbies might be making your back pain worse, aging your bones and joints faster than normal and slowing your healing, and how addressing all of these areas is the key to creating a nearly superhuman spine.

You'll understand exactly how your back works, what makes it strong, and what makes it weak. In other words, you'll know how to use your spine properly so that it lasts your entire life. It doesn't matter if you're in your twenties or your eighties – if you follow the instructions in this book, you'll have less pain and get more use out of your neck and back.

This book does not go into great detail regarding the anatomy and physiology of the spine and different musculoskeletal conditions. Nor does it provide extensive information on why different treatments provide the results they do. Many books are already available that provide such information. Instead, this book was meant to be written like an actual instruction manual. In a manner similar to the manual that came with your car or home appliances, I've striven to provide simple instructions for proper spinal use, relevant warnings to avoid disuse, and troubleshooting instructions when things go wrong.

# 2

# The Emergency Back Pain Checklist

If you are having any of the following, consult an emergency physician immediately:

- **Radiating pain down your arms, legs, or into your face or jaw.**
- **Loss of bowel or bladder control.**
- **Dizziness, nausea, vertigo, or vomiting associated with your pain.**
- **Intractable pain down your arms, legs, or into your face.**
- **Loss of muscle function in your arms, legs, or face.**
- **Loss of sensation in your arms, legs, or face.**
- **If you feel as though you are having a medical emergency.**
- **If you feel in any way that you need to see a doctor immediately.**
- **Rate your pain on a scale from 1-10, with 1 being no pain and 10 being pain so severe that you can't walk or move without help. If you can't move or walk without help, consult an emergency physician immediately.**

1. For pain occurring within the last 48-72 hours, using an ice pack on the area of pain is generally the best option. A store-bought ice pack or ice cubes and a little water in a Ziploc freezer bag placed within a pillowcase to prevent contacting the skin directly will suffice. The pack must remain on the area of pain for 15 minutes, then off for 2 hours, repeated as needed.
2. If you choose to take any over-the-counter pain medications, follow the label recommendations.
3. If you feel a cane or brace is needed for support and/or pain relief, do not hesitate to use either or both.
4. Do not get a massage for the first week following the onset of sudden back or neck pain.
5. Do not use heating pads or packs for the first three days following the onset of your pain.
6. If you shower within the first three days following the onset of pain, do not let the hot water flow for prolonged periods over the area of pain. Get in, shower, and get out.
7. Avoid sitting for prolonged periods. If you must sit, only sit for approximately 15 minutes before standing and either gently walking or standing and gently rocking in place for 3-5 minutes.
8. If you must sit, try to use the tallest chair available to sit on. This will minimize the pain experienced and muscle effort needed to stand later on.
9. If your bed is generally soft and you have a firmer bed available to sleep on in your home, try using the firmer bed if you can tolerate it.
10. Avoid lying down for prolonged periods (greater than one hour) except for sleeping at night. When lying down to rest (i.e., not when going to bed at night), try to gently

change positions slightly (bending the knees, bending one knee and then the other, gently moving to one side, then the other, etc.) while lying to prevent your muscles from getting too stiff.

11. Once three days have passed from the onset of pain and the pain intensity is starting to reduce, heat is generally safe to use. The frequency of use is the same as with ice: 15 minutes on, and 2 hours off. Be careful to use heat that is significantly warm but not so hot as to burn or cause skin damage.

12. If, during the first three days following the onset of pain, the pain is not reducing in intensity at all from a 1–10 scale, or if any of the symptoms in Step 1 begin to occur, consult a physician immediately.

13. If after three days, your pain is reducing in intensity and none of the symptoms at the start of this checklist are being experienced, continue home care instructions and consider a chiropractic evaluation to determine the extent of your injury and to develop a plan for full healing.

14. If you should aggravate your pain at any time during the first week after the onset, take stock of yourself and determine if you are feeling any of the symptoms at the start of this checklist. If so, consult an emergency physician immediately. If not, jump to Steps 1–13.

ADDITIONAL NOTES:

· Pineapple is a good natural anti-inflammatory nutrition source, due to the bromelain enzyme found within. If you are currently taking any prescription medications, confirm with your doctor that pineapple is safe to eat before consuming. Fresh-cut or canned pineapple (in water, not syrup) are both good choices.

- Drink plenty of water. Your spasming muscles with be burning through your body's water reserves in their attempt to stay contracted and keep you protected. Drinking enough water will help reduce unnecessary muscle cramping.
- There are many OTC roll-ons and topicals available at drugstores and pharmacies that contain lidocaine, an anesthetic commonly used to treat pain. Aspercreme and Icy-Hot both have products that contain lidocaine. These may help alleviate pain that is more superficial than deep. If used, be sure to follow the label instructions.

# 3

# Understand Your Back, Understand Your Pain

I want you to take a moment and imagine something. Imagine you've been given twenty four wooden blocks. Your task is to stack those blocks up in such a way that they don't sway or topple over. It's a task that takes a little bit of effort, but one the average person should be able to do without huge difficulty.

Let's assume for a minute that you've accomplished this task. You stacked up all 24 blocks and there they sit in front of you, perfectly balanced.

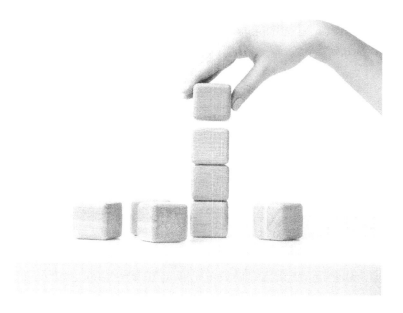

Now, I'm going to make it a little harder.

I'm going to now take a saw to those 24 blocks. I'm going to shave off some wood here and some wood there, and I'm going to change the shape of each of these blocks from a simple cube into what amounts to a three-dimensional jigsaw puzzle piece for each.

Now I'm going to give you the same task. Assemble these 24 wooden pieces into a stack that is able to balance without falling over. Yes, I know, this task just got infinitely harder. However, to make it easier, I'm going to give you a bag of 100 rubber bands to help you make these pieces stick together. Alright, get to work.

Let's assume you're able to balance this tower on a table without it falling over.

I'm about to make things harder.

I want you to arrange the wooden blocks in such a way that the stack now resembles a letter "S" instead of a straight vertical stack. Be sure that, once you've done this, the stack is still able to balance on the table without falling over.

Let's make things even harder.

I want you to take a 100-pound weight and place it on the top of the stack and balance it in such a way that it doesn't fall over.

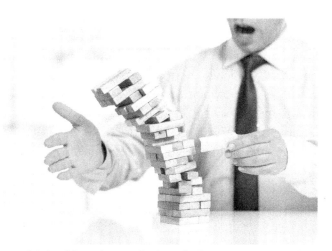

*Balancing multiple objects in gravity is a challenge. Our spine does it every second of every day.*

Impossible, right? Pretty much.

Let's take it up another notch. Take the stack of 24 puzzle-piece shaped wooden blocks with the 100-pound weight plate and balance it in the palm of your hand. Feel free to move your hand around in order to make sure the stack maintains its balance and doesn't fall over.

Are you finding this task difficult yet?

Good. I describe this exercise in detail for one reason...*to get you to understand how your spine is able to function every day, allowing you to walk, run, bend, twist, and allow you to live your life without collapsing to the ground.*

Your spine is basically a stack of 24 irregularly shaped jigsaw puzzle pieces, held together with a stack of rubber bands which represent the muscles and ligaments that hold your bones together and make them move. A healthy spine maintains an S-shaped curve when viewed from the side that bends forward in the neck (cervical) region, back in the mid back (thoracic) region, and forward again in the lower back (lumbar) region. These curves provide shock absorption and provide movement in virtually any direction, which lets us work, play sports, and do almost anything physical that we can think of. When viewed from the front or back, this stack of bones should make a perfectly straight line.

**Vertebral Column: Lateral view**

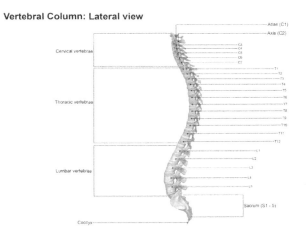

**Vertebral column: Posterior view**

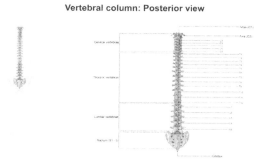

This system of interlocking vertebrae also make a bony tube that the spinal cord travels through. At each vertebral level, nerve roots branch off from the spinal cord and run to various parts of the body, monitoring and controlling our muscles, joints, and organs. This is the other reason the spine is so important. Not only will problems with spinal balance lead to potential back pain and degeneration, irritation or pressure on the nerve roots exiting the spine can lead to potential long-term health conditions that may be difficult to treat with standard medical means.

Thus, the shape of the spine created by the particular alignment of our vertebrae is the single most important aspect that will determine whether a person will develop chronic back pain, let alone other medical symptoms. Proper spinal shape will lead to proper spinal function and the ability to bear the forces that we encounter on a daily basis with minimal degeneration. In contrast, improper spinal shape will lead to premature degeneration and increase the risk for injury and pain. A person

15

with an improper spinal shape who is suffering greater than average forces on their spine will be in an even worse situation, as an abnormal spinal shape will wear out much faster than a normal one.

The nature of the spinal structures requires that different forces be applied to make a change from an abnormal spine to a normal spine. Hard bones can be moved by hand in order to help joints move better, but muscles and ligaments need forces applied over a longer time in order to make a lasting, permanent change to the overall shape of the spine.

Consider a rubber band. Stretch it for a moment and it returns to its normal shape. But, stretch a rubber band around a basketball and leave it for a week. When you remove the rubber band from the ball, you will notice it has taken on a new, permanent shape, thanks to the stretching forces applied to it for an extended period of time. Making permanent changes to the spine via the muscles and ligaments requires consistent, targeted pressure in a similar manner.

When it comes to fixing back pain, the shape of the spine is what matters most. Of secondary importance are the types and duration of forces placed on the spine. Thus, treatment that covers restoration of spinal shape and movement and also removes or modifies any daily position or activity that places undue pressure on the spine will get the best results.

# 4

# Meet Your Back

## The Bones

Your spinal bones (vertebrae) are the literal "bricks" that make up the building known as your spine. However, their design is perfect when it comes to supporting the weight of your body. Each vertebrae has a hard, bony outer covering called "cortical" bone, while the interior of the vertebrae looks like spider webs. This weblike structural design is called "cancellous" bone. The purpose behind this design is ingenious in its simplicity. Having different projections of bone in many directions within the vertebrae allows it to support the weight of the body and forces placed on it from any direction, while still remaining lightweight.

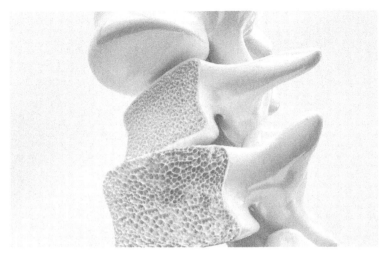

*Cross section of a vertebrae showing web-like cancellous bone*

The joints, or "facets", are the structures that allow each vertebrae to fit together. Each spinal bone rests on the facets of the one below it in a manner similar to dinner plates stacked together, instead of interlocking like Lego pieces. The facet joint design allows for support but also allows for enough flexible movement to allow us to do the things we do, but restricts unsafe movement that could cause injury.

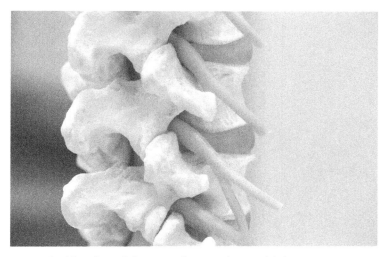

*Interlocking facet joints are shown, along with bony processes.*

If you look at a vertebrae, you'll notice several points of bone projecting out in different directions. These are known as "processes" and they are points where muscles and ligaments attach to the vertebrae.

## The Muscles

Back muscles are divided into two groups: intrinsic and extrinsic. The extrinsic muscles, such as the latissimus dorsi, trapezius, rhomboids and others, are commonly known because our gym workouts usually involve working these muscle regions. However, the intrinsic spinal muscles are the ones most commonly affected during a back injury, and as such, will be our focus here.

19

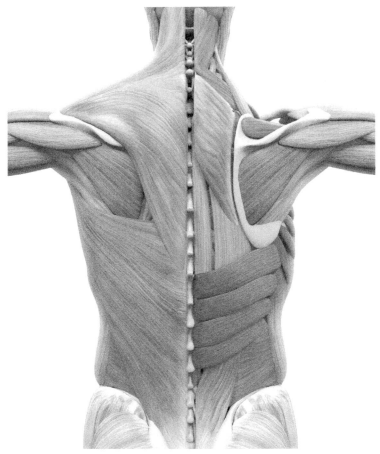

*Extrinsic muscles shown left of the spine, while intrinsic muscles shown at right above.*

The intrinsic back muscles have three layers - superficial, intermediate, and deep. These muscles help you balance and move your spinal bones. The back and sides of the neck are where the superficial intrinsic muscles are found, where they control movement of the head and neck in nearly all directions. The intermediate intrinsic muscles are found on each side of the vertebrae, running from the back of the skull down to the base of the spine. They control extension (backward bending) of the spine and help maintain normal spinal position. The deep intrinsic muscles are the smallest spinal muscles, often running from a single vertebrae to another in some areas. These muscles also help manage spinal position but also act as monitors, measuring the amount of stretch and pressure placed on the spine at any given moment. When they sense abnormal forces being placed on the spine, they trigger muscle spasms that lock up vertebral motion to prevent further injury. This is the feeling you feel when your back is "out."

## The Ligaments

Several layers of ligaments surround the vertebrae and provide stability throughout our full range of movement. The anterior longitudinal ligament connects the front of each vertebral body from the top of the neck to the bottom of the back, while the posterior longitudinal ligament connects the back of each vertebral body from top to bottom. These long ligaments act as stabilizers, limiting excessive forward or backward movement that could injure the spinal column. The supraspinous ligament also runs from the top of the neck to the bottom of the back. This ligament connects the rearmost portion of each vertebrae known as the spinous processes, which are the bony projections you can feel when you run your fingers over your spine.

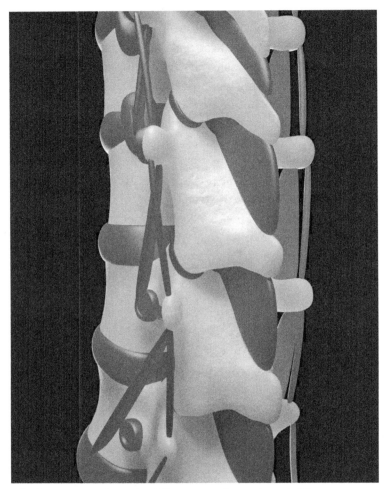

*Various connective spinal ligaments shown in red. Discs are seen between the vertebral bodies.*

The ligamentum flavum runs the entire length of the spine, covering the rear portion of the vertebral ring that the spinal cord passes through. This ligament connects each vertebrae and helps restore normal spinal position after bending, in addition to protecting the spinal cord.

Additional small ligaments called capsular ligaments connect the vertebrae at their joints while the interspinous ligaments connect each vertebrae between the spinous processes.

## The Discs

The intervertebral discs are a true feat of biological engineering. Each disc that sits between your spinal bones has three parts – an inner nucleus pulposus, concentric rings of collagen called the annulus fibrosus, and an outer cartilage cover that connects the disc to the vertebrae above and below it.

# THE STRUCTURE OF THE VERTEBRA

## (Top view)

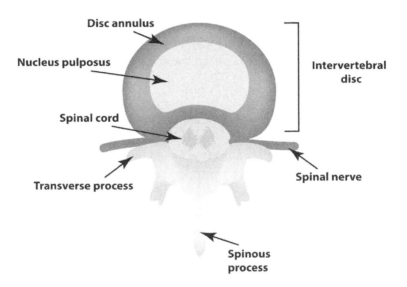

Disc annulus

Nucleus pulposus

Intervertebral disc

Spinal cord

Transverse process

Spinal nerve

Spinous process

The nucleus pulposus sits in the center of the disc and is mostly water mixed with the same type of collagen found in other joints of the body. The design of the nucleus pulposus plays a major role in the spine's ability to move and withstand pressure.

The annulus fibrosus rings within the disc are also made of collagen, and each ring's fibers are oriented in the opposite direction of its adjacent rings. This design allows the disc to maintain strength in each direction of twist, since there are

24

fibers simultaneously allowing and restricting rotation in each direction.

Healthy discs are also important to nerve and joint function. The height of a healthy disc is what provides the space between each vertebrae for the spinal nerves to pass between. The spinal joints are also spaced correctly when the discs are a healthy height and shape. Degenerating, thinning discs cause the vertebrae to rest closer to each other than they should, which pushes joint surfaces closer together and causes the dull, achy pain that so many back pain patients feel.

# 5

# How To Sit

The act of sitting, while seemingly benign, places a great deal of stress on the front of the spinal bones and the discs. Ordinarily, the discs and vertebral bodies of the lumbar vertebrae are meant to carry approximately ⅓ of the weight placed on them, with the remaining ⅔ being supported by each of the spinal joints. In the sitting position, the lumbar spine flexes forward, placing 100 percent of the stress on the vertebral body and disc. If this position is maintained for a brief period, there are no damaging long-term effects. However, if this position is held for long periods of time at regular intervals, this excessive pressure causes the discs to wear out prematurely and contributes to premature arthritic degeneration of the vertebral body.

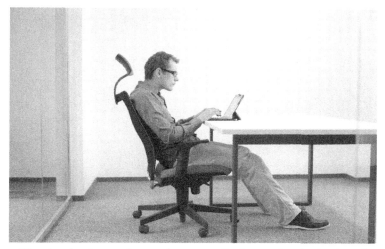

*The classic, slumped seated posture. Bad news for the back and neck.*

The proper sitting position is to be sitting forward at the edge of your chair with your knees lower than your hips. Your feet should be resting underneath your hips, if possible. This position allows your pelvis to rock slightly forward and your spine to more easily maintain a proper, upright position. The spinal joints, discs, and vertebral bodies are evenly sharing the weight of the upper body when sitting this way, which also reduces the likelihood of premature spinal aging and disc degeneration.

27

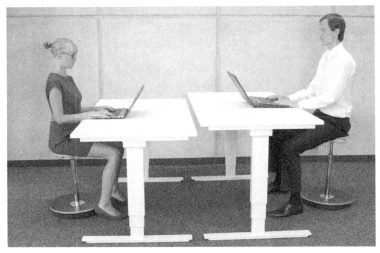

*Proper, healthy sitting posture. Note the knees are lower than the hips, and both use their eyes to look down instead of bending their head forward excessively.*

After sitting for any 15 minute period, you should get up and walk for 3-5 minutes. Anyone with a job that requires sitting should try to follow this schedule as frequently as possible. If you can't walk for 3-5 minutes, standing at your desk and doing some simple stretches, spinal twists, or rocking your hips side to side will also do.

A good alternative is to sit in the position mentioned above for 5 minutes, then switch to a full seated position, which is completely back in your chair with your spine resting against the seatback. Sit this way for 5 minutes and then switch back to the forward seated position on the edge of the chair. After 15 minutes, get up and walk/stretch for 3-5 minutes as described. This will also help minimize unwanted stress on the lower back.

# 6

# How To Stand

Thanks to recent media coverage of the dangers of prolonged sitting, standing desks and standing work environments have become the new work ergonomic trend. However, standing at work does not come without risks. Studies are now showing that people who stand for long periods of time at work are often developing leg swelling along with lower back and leg pain. I know what you're thinking – *"I can't sit, I can't stand...what am I supposed to do?"*

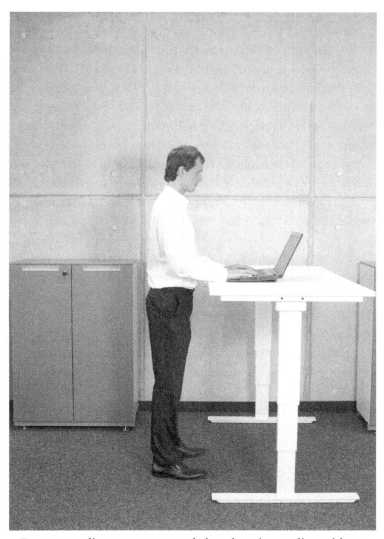

*Proper standing posture at work, but chronic standing without movement can often be as damaging as chronic sitting. Movement is the medicine.*

The problem is not that a person sits or stands at work. The problem arises when all someone does at work is sit or stand. Taking frequent breaks to change body positions is necessary to blunt the effects of prolonged sitting or standing. If you must stand at work, have a seat for a couple of minutes after you've stood for 15 minutes. If you're unable to take a seat, the next best alternative is to take a brief walk for a few minutes after each 15 minutes of standing. If your job requires you to do nothing but stand and walk all day, you will still feel the effects of this activity over time, and your only choices are to make sure your footwear is comfortable enough to last you the entire day or consider alternate job options.

I know the latter choice sounds extreme, but when you consider that the quality of life you have later depends on what you do now, switching to a different job that doesn't wear on your body so much will pay off over the long run. You'll feel better now, which will keep you productive at work, and you'll feel less wear and tear later, which will allow you to enjoy your time off and/or retirement to a greater extent.

If a job switch isn't an option, get good footwear, take breaks when you can, and see your chiropractor and massage therapist for regular checkups to keep your joints as mobile as possible.

# 7

# How To Sleep

Getting a good night's sleep is essential for your back to heal up from the day's traumas and return to normal. However, the only way to ensure you get a good 7-9 hours of sleep is for your back to be comfortable while sleeping. A painful, stiff, or sore back will make you miserable all night long, and you can bet you'll feel the same way come sunrise.

Getting your back comfortable and ready for a night's sleep starts with your sleeping position. The best sleeping position is 1) on your side with your knees bent, and 2) on your back, with or without a pillow under your knees (not important if you can do without it.) These two positions put the least amount of stress on your back when sleeping. You should try to make either or both of these positions the norm for your sleeping routine to ensure your back has the best chance to recover from the day's activities.

Having the right mattress will also ensure your back stays comfortable while you sleep. I get asked all the time what kind of mattress is the best, and the answer is: **the best mattress for you is the one that is as firm as possible BUT still comfortable FOR YOU to sleep on.** A firmer mattress will keep your spine in proper position as you sleep. A softer mattress will bow under your weight during the night, essentially forcing you to sleep as if you were in a hammock. Sleeping in a bowed position will do the same thing to your back as if you walked around leaning to one side for several hours a day. This is easily avoided by taking the time to find a mattress with the perfect blend of firmness and comfort.

CORRECT AND INCORRECT SLEEPING POSITION

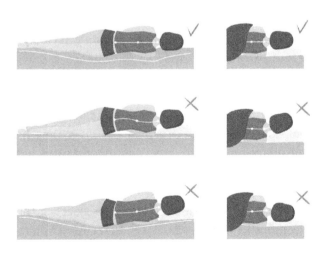

Shopping for the right mattress should be an all-day affair. You can't possibly know whether a particular mattress you try out for five minutes in the store will still feel the same after a month of sleeping on it. When trying out mattresses, be prepared to lay on a possible mattress choice for 45 minutes to an hour before deciding whether you like it or not. Kick your shoes off and get comfy. As you lay there, grab your cell phone and start scrolling through your apps, just like you'd do in bed. You'll have a much better chance of picking the right firmness by "living in it" for an hour and seeing how it really feels.

The only mattress brand I have ever recommended is the Sleep Number Bed. It has an adjustable mattress that has a hundred different firmness settings, making it effortless to find the firmness setting that works for you. It's like buying 100 different mattresses and finding which one matches you perfectly. The Sleep Number bed even has dual adjustability for each side of the mattress, which means you and your partner can have different firmness settings that work for both of you, ensuring you both sleep your best each night. You can find out more at sleepnumber.com.

## How do I find the right pillow to prevent neck pain?

When it comes to finding the right pillow for your neck, the biggest factor you should concern yourself with is the size of the pillow. Buying a pillow is like buying a pair of shoes. It doesn't matter how affordable or expensive your favorite pair of shoes were when you got them. What matters is you got them in a size that fits you so they would be comfortable when you wore them.

When trying to determine the right size pillow, a measurement should be taken from the bony point of your skull just behind your ear to the outer edge of your shoulder bone (humerus). This measurement is the approximate measurement that your pillow should be when compressed by the weight of your head while laying on your side. This measurement will be different for almost everybody. But this measurement is important to make sure that when sleeping on your side in bed, your head is lifted properly enough to stay in line with your spine and not stretched downward or upward too much. This is probably the single most overlooked reason for neck pain, headaches, and the carpal-tunnel-syndrome-like hand numbness that some feel when they wake up in the morning.

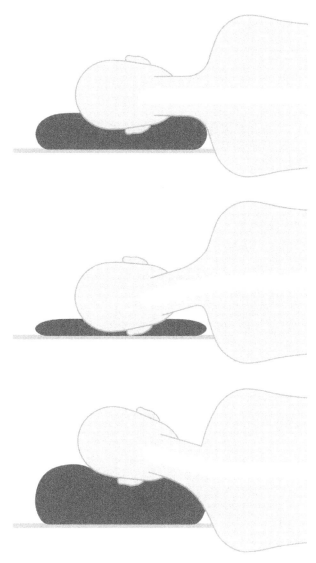

*The right size pillow will keep your head where it needs to be all night – in line with the rest of your spine.*

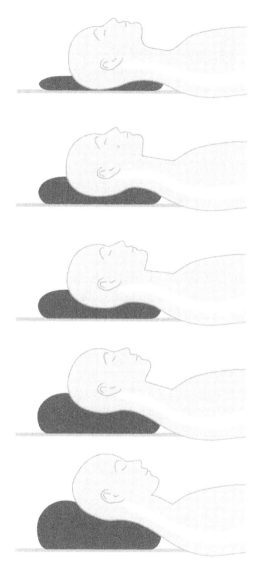

*The higher the pillow, the higher the chance of developing neck stiffness, numbness, and tingling in the hands when you wake up.*

There are only a few companies that make pillows based on size. The company I have referred patients to most is Therapeutica. On their website, you can review how the pillow works and also are shown how to take a measurement at home to determine what size pillow is the proper size for you. Some pillow company websites have generic information stating if you wake up with pain, your pillow might be the wrong size and you should get a different one — but they don't give any information about how to find the right size, nor do they sell pillows in a variety of different sizes to make sure that a person can find the right one for them.

In my opinion, the best place to start is with Therapeutica. Their pillow is designed for back and side sleepers, which are the two best positions to avoid neck pain. When you're laying on your back, the Therapeutica pillow properly supports the curve of your neck, cradles your head, and allows for support on the upper back. When you roll to either side, a Therapeutica pillow sized correctly will keep your head in line with the rest of your body, which prevents undue neck strain and nerve pressure that can cause hand numbness and tingling. The right size pillow will give you a better night's sleep, allow damaged neck muscles and joints to heal faster, and make you a healthier, happier person.

# 8

# How To Bend and Lift

Bending has likely caused more back injuries than any other common daily movement, with lifting a close second. Our back is designed to bend forward and backward within a reasonable range of motion, but in the current age of long commutes, desk jobs, and TV show binge watching, our weakened backs may not always be ready to offer full bending range of motion at a moment's notice. Thus, "protected bending" is the best way to prevent unnecessary back injuries.

- When bending forward to pick up an object off the floor or ground, place one hand on your knee as you bend at the knees and then use your other hand to pick up the object.
- To lift something heavy, get someone to help and place your hands under the object and move your chest and hips as close as possible to the object.
- Straighten your back up and **breathe out continuously** as you engage your legs to lift yourself and the object off the ground. **Continue breathing out** until your legs are fully

extended and you are standing upright.

· Walk carefully until you're ready to set the object down, and then straighten your back and **breathe out continuously** as you bend your knees and lower yourself and the object to the ground.

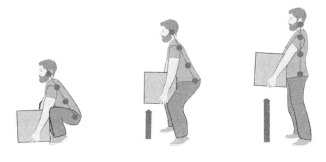

*The right way to pick up a heavy object. To set it down, simply follow these steps in reverse.*

In instances where your back is already injured and you need to pick up something off the floor, place one foot in front of the other and use the forward leg to support your body weight as you bend forward carefully. Obviously, do not lift more than small amounts of weight when your back is injured.

# 9

# How To Carry

When carrying objects that run the risk of causing injury to your back, it's important to keep the objects as close to the mid-line of your body as possible. Suitcases, buckets, baby carriers — we often carry objects like these to the side of our body, which can pull our back posture off to one side and cause potential back strain. When you have no choice but to carry items like these, switch the carrying side every few minutes so that the muscles and joints on both sides of your back can share the load.

The side-switching tactic can even be used when doing simple housework or yard work. When I sweep my driveway or even my kitchen floor, I sweep about a half dozen times in one direction before switching the broom to my other hand and sweeping with it another half dozen times or so before switching back. This process works for shovels, rakes, squeegees, pool cleaning tools, or any implement that requires the use of both arms. Switching positions frequently will ease the burden on your joints and muscles and cause your fewer problems for your back.

# 10

# How To Exercise

Exercising is one of the best things you can do to keep your back healthy your entire life. However, exercising with poor form or overloading your back too much can have devastating effects that can stay with you for decades.

If you're working out with weights or plan to, the exercises you should be extremely cautious with (or avoid altogether) are squats and deadlifts. If you decide to do these exercises, make sure you pay strict attention to your form and use a weight that you can absolutely handle that doesn't cause your back or legs to shake when performing the exercise. And don't feel as though you're cheating yourself out of a good workout if you decide to skip squats or deadlifts. There are several other good back and leg workouts that don't carry the same risk of injury but will still give you a good workout "burn" that will last for days. Examples include leg curls, lunges, box jumps, and others. Talk to a personal trainer for exercise substitutions as needed.

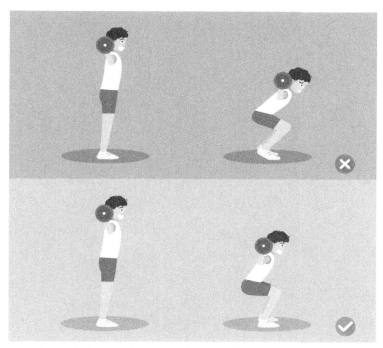

*Failing to follow perfect squat form with reasonable weight will lead to injury.*

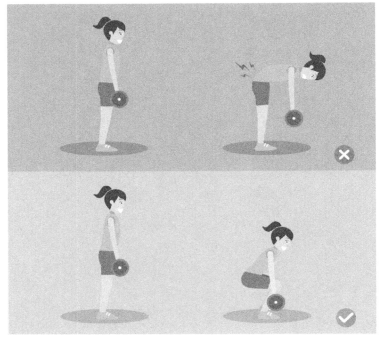

*Failing to follow perfect deadlift form with reasonable weight will also lead to injury.*

A few additional exercise tips:

- When doing back hyperextensions, avoid bending too far backwards at the end of the motion. Stop when your back is in line with your pelvis and legs.
- If you perform leg presses, keep your head back against the back pad when pushing and lowering the weight.
- Breathe out in one slow, steady continuous breath when lifting and lowering weight.

- Make sure you're working each body part one time per week.
- Get adequate rest, water, and nutrition to support your body's recovery from weight or cardio training.

Another factor to consider when weight training is reaching a maximum limit. I routinely see patients who work out regularly but come in with back injuries because they are always trying to push heavier and heavier weights and hit "new goals." The problem with this philosophy is that we, as human beings, can only eat so much nutrition in a day. We can only drink so much fluid. We can only sleep so many hours each day. If all these factors are finite but we continue to push heavier and heavier weight in an attempt to reach new personal weight lifting goals, we are simply begging for an injury, and a possibly devastating one at that.

You need to determine what amount of weight (within reason) you want to bench press, or squat, or curl, or whatever, and once you hit that goal, you stay within that general range and maintain your fitness level using that amount of weight. Doing so will prevent unnecessary injuries, allowing your workouts to be more productive and less damaging.

As far as the best kind of workouts, nothing beats swimming for cardio. Swimming is the perfect, low impact cardio workout that anyone with access to a pool can do. A good alternative to cardio is the elliptical machine, which also provides a great workout with minimal stress to the major joints of the body. If the elliptical machine is too boring or doesn't seem to fit you, another option is a mountain climber machine, which is what I use for my cardio workout. It works the entire body instead of simply the lower body, and it gets your heart rate up in a hurry so you're not killing extra time. Plus, it's safe and fairly easy on the joints, but people with knee injuries may not be able to go at a very hard pace due to the nature of the motion performed on the machine.

# II

# Troubleshooting Your Neck and Back Pain

*What To Do When You*
*Sit, Stand, Walk, Sleep, Bend, Lift, Carry, or Exercise*
*Incorrectly*

# 11

## Determine The Cause

In most back pain cases, there is a definite event or injury that preceded your pain. You may remember such an event or injury within the last day or two if you've developed sudden discomfort. If you're unable to move without pain in the same way you did when the injury happened, it's very likely that your pain was mostly or completely caused by that event.

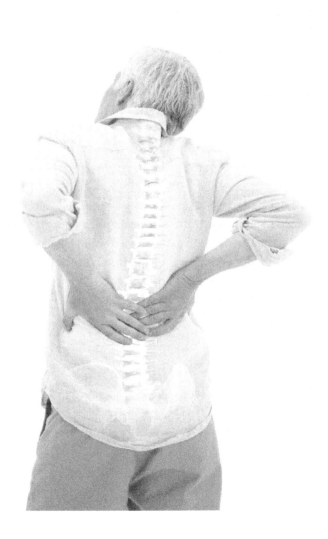

It's also likely your pain wasn't caused by one specific event you can remember, but may be the result of several days of overuse, stress, or repetitive movements building up within your musculoskeletal system. These triggers can compound daily until a seemingly simple task - such as bending over to tie your shoes or pick up something off the floor - causes your back to lock up and go into severe spasm. In cases like these, the movements or body positions you've put yourself through over the last few days that caused your pain may not be easily identifiable. You may have the same routine with work and home life day in and day out. In these situations, a doctor who knows how to ask the right questions can help you pinpoint which habits, body positions, or activities are guilty of slowly tearing you down and weakening your back.

Once you have identified the cause of your pain, it's much easier to treat and make recommendations that help keep future occurrences of pain to a minimum. However, RELY ON AN EXPERT such as your doctor to help you determine which activities or positions to avoid and how to manage the healing process. And as hard as it may be, try to avoid becoming a "Google doctor" in an attempt to diagnose and treat yourself. If you absolutely can't keep yourself off the internet, bring your ideas and questions to your doctor and let them help you make sense of it all.

# 12

# Using Ice and Heat Properly

Whenever you have a sudden injury or flare-up of pain, always use ice for the first two to three days. Ice works faster and more effectively than over-the-counter medication because it goes to work immediately at the site of pain, as opposed to medication which can take up to 30 minutes for the effect to circulate through your body. **The timing of ice use should be as follows: 15 minutes on, two hours off.** Repeat as needed or as long as you have time.

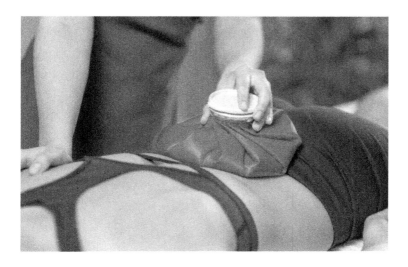

There are varying stages of sensation you'll feel when ice is applied to your body. They are cold, burning, aching, and finally, numbness. You'll feel these different stages as the ice goes to work. As long as the ice pack you're using is not directly touching your skin, do your best to grin and bear the burning and aching until the numbness stage is reached.

Do not use heat during this time period. Heat will only com-pound any macro- or micro-swelling and make you feel worse. Yes, heat does feel good when it is applied, but the next day you'll feel like you were hit with a bat if you use it when the swelling process is still active.

Continue using ice until two or three days have passed. At this time, the inflammation period has usually subsided and it's okay to start using heat at the same frequency and duration you used the ice – 15 minutes on, two hours off.

<u>When in doubt about which therapy to go with, use ice.</u> There are wrong times to use heat, but there's never a wrong time to use ice. Don't deviate from the timing of 15 on, two hours off, either, whether using heat or ice.

# 13

# Stretching For Healing

In the not too distant past, doctors routinely prescribed bed rest to their patients whenever they suffered back pain. It was assumed that this period of rest was beneficial in helping the injured tissues heal properly to avoid a recurrence of pain.

Today, doctors have learned a great deal about the negative effects of bed rest during back pain episodes. For back pain not caused by fractures or freshly herniated discs, bed rest has taken a back seat in favor of active movement, light stretching, and various physical modalities such as chiropractic, massage, and physical therapy. We now know that resting muscles and joints that have sustained certain types of injuries actually makes them less likely to repair and come back stronger. In these cases, muscles and joints need movement to ensure the proper alignment of muscle fibers during healing and to prepare these healing tissues for the forces they will have to endure once back to normal. This "movement" can come in the form of any of the modalities mentioned previously.

This does not mean that bed rest is off the table as a recommended form of therapy. Cases of severe, acute back pain that makes any movement impossible requires rest for the first day or two to allow swelling and inflammation to subside. These kinds of cases are best treated by obtaining x-rays or MRIs to determine specific causes of pain, and thus, to determine the best form of treatment.

Light stretching through a reasonable range of motion after a back injury is recommended to help the muscles and joint tissues heal more flexibly. Don't push yourself too far into the point of pain; instead, stop once you feel slight discomfort or resistance. As you heal, your range of motion will increase day by day until it returns to normal.

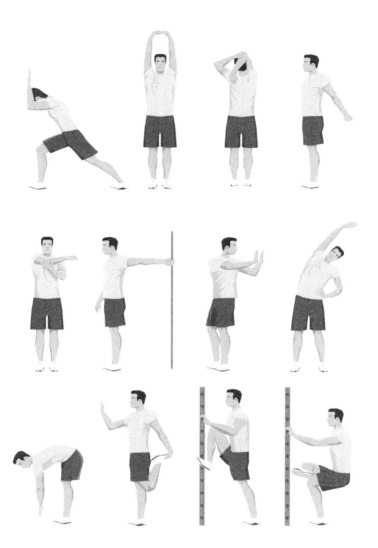

*Stretching while you heal is virtually always good, but don't do too much too soon.*

# 14

# Should You Take Pain Pills or Medicine For Your Pain?

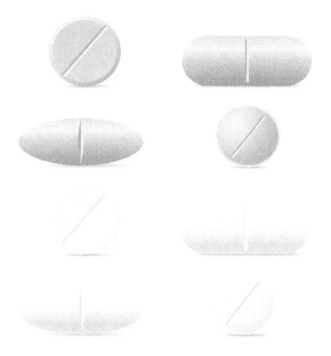

Anyone who's in pain should try to get relief as quickly as possible. We all have busy lives that we need to get back to as soon as possible. Pain medication can often help reduce your misery enough to function, but is it the best choice for long term pain relief.

In my opinion, pain medicine should definitely be used in the early stages of pain in order to simply provide relief while you heal. It also helps lower the pain enough for you to begin treatment to alleviate the cause of the pain. Having a lower pain experience makes it easier for you to start doing exercises or stretches or other treatments to correct the cause of your pain.

You need to make sure that you follow your medical doctor's instructions as it pertains to any medication that you're given. And obviously, If you decide to use any over the counter medications for pain relief, be sure to follow the label instructions.

Some people don't want to take pain medication because they're concerned about side effects. They don't want medication side effects or they feel the side effects are worse than the pain they're feeling. Some patients are afraid of getting addicted to pain medication. While these are valid concerns, your other option is to use other non-medication pain relieving methods for pain relief that have zero side effects and no risk of addiction. In the end, be sure to educate yourself on all the available choices, speak to your doctor, and choose the one that will allow you to get on with corrective treatment as soon as possible.

# 15

# When To Use a Back or Neck Brace

There are times when a back or neck brace is absolutely necessary. Those times are usually after an accident when there is so much soft tissue damage that any movement will make the injury significantly worse. Examples include motor vehicle accidents or severe sports injuries.

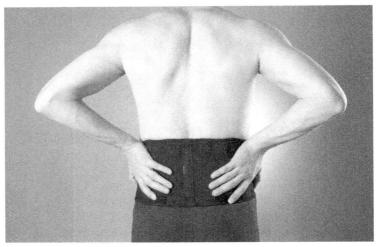

*Back braces can be extremely helpful, but be prepared to wean off of it as you heal.*

However, the majority of the time, most back and neck pains do not require a back or neck brace in order to get better. In fact, prolonged use of braces leads to weakening of the spinal muscles whose job it is to stabilize and move the neck and back as needed throughout your day. Letting those muscles lose their strength is the fastest way to increase the likelihood of more injuries down the road.

There is an exception to every rule. There are often times when a patient's pain is so severe that a brace may be necessary to simply give their overworked muscles a break for a few days. I have had success in those isolated cases with braces, but those patients are diagnosed on a case-by-case basis. In general, most patients should avoid braces unless their doctor has prescribed one. And even in those cases, the brace should come off as soon as medically possible.

# 16

## When Should You See a Chiropractor, PT, Medical Doctor, or Massage Therapist?

When you have back pain, it's hard to know sometimes which doctor to go to first. If you're having severe pain that is preventing you from performing regular life tasks like standing or walking, your best bet is to go to an ER or urgent care for the first line of pain relief. There, they will provide medication that will take a measure of the pain down and possibly do imaging studies to rule out more serious conditions.

Once your back pain is a more manageable level or you've gone to urgent care and ruled out any medical contraindications to treatment, you should see a chiropractor next. I say this because medical doctors often refer to physical therapists for pain relief, but if a person's spine is out of balance due to poor posture or some other musculoskeletal anomaly, a chiropractor will be the best choice to develop a treatment plan to get your spinal structure back to ideal normal as soon as possible.

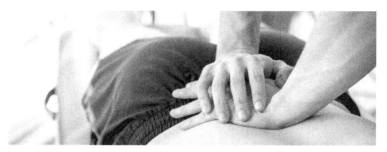

*A chiropractic adjustment is one of the most effective means of treating back pain available.*

According to the American Chiropractic Association, the following facts are known:

- 31 million Americans experience low back pain at any given time.1
- Worldwide, back pain is the single leading cause of disability, preventing many people from engaging in work as well as other everyday activities.2
- Back pain is one of the most common reasons for missed work. One-half of all working Americans admit to having back pain symptoms each year.3
- Back pain accounts for more than 264 million lost work days in one year—that's two work days for every full-time worker in the country.4
- Experts estimate that up to 80% of the population will experience back pain at some time in their lives.5
- Back pain can affect people of all ages, from adolescents to

the elderly.5
- Back pain is the third most common reason for visits to the doctor's office, behind skin disorders and osteoarthritis/joint disorders.6
- Most cases of back pain are mechanical or non-organic—meaning they are not caused by serious conditions, such as inflammatory arthritis, infection, fracture or cancer.7
- Most people with low back pain recover, however recurrence is common and for a small percentage of people the condition will become chronic and disabling.7
- Worldwide, years lived with disability caused by low back pain have increased by 54% between 1990 and 2015.7
- Low-back pain costs Americans at least $50 billion in health care costs each year8—add in lost wages and decreased productivity and that figure easily rises to more than $100 billion.9

In the midst of our nation's opioid overuse epidemic, spinal manipulation is receiving greater attention as a non-drug means of providing pain relief. It lowers pain (while also lowering the need for medication in many cases), improves physical therapy outcomes, and requires very few passive forms of treatment, such as bed rest.10

A growing body of research supports spinal manipulation as a means of maintaining proper spinal function and reducing pain. Again, according to the American Chiropractic Association:

- After an extensive study of all available care for low back problems, the federal Agency for Health Care Policy and

Research (now the Agency for Health Care Research and Quality) recommended that low back pain sufferers choose the most conservative care first. And it recommended spinal manipulation as the only safe and effective, drugless form of initial professional treatment for acute low back problems in adults.11

· A well-respected review of the evidence in the *Annals of Internal Medicine* pointed to chiropractic care as one of the major non-drug therapies considered effective for acute and chronic low back pain.12

· According to an article in the medical journal *Spine*, there is strong evidence that spinal manipulation for back pain is just as effective as a combination of medical care and exercise, and there is moderate evidence that it is just as effective as prescription NSAIDS combined with exercise. 13

· An article in the *Journal of the American Medical Association* suggested chiropractic care as an option for people suffering from low back pain—and noted that surgery is usually not needed and should only be tried if other therapies fail.14

· More recently, the results of a clinical trial published in *JAMA Network Open* showed that chiropractic care combined with usual medical care for low back pain provides greater pain relief and a greater reduction in disability than medical care alone. The study, which featured 750 active-duty members of the military, is one of the largest comparative effectiveness trials between usual medical care and chiropractic care ever conducted.15

For many patients suffering from back pain, spinal manipulation can be very effective at reducing pain and improving function. However, the majority of patients seeking relief will

69

need more than just manipulation to completely heal and reduce recurrences of pain. The positions we place our backs in throughout the day, the demands we place on our muscles and joints, and the complete history of our back injuries and damages will determine what extra types of treatment will be necessary to get better. Patients whose spines need a comprehensive plan of treatment — which includes not only treatment for pain relief, but also treatment for pain prevention — will get the best results because everything that is making their back worse is addressed, making them almost resistant to pain and degeneration.

Physical therapists are good at getting function restored, but you can't have ideal function without ideal structure. It's best to let the chiropractor do their thing and possibly even co-treat with a PT, although many modalities that are done in a PT office can also be done at home with a little instruction.

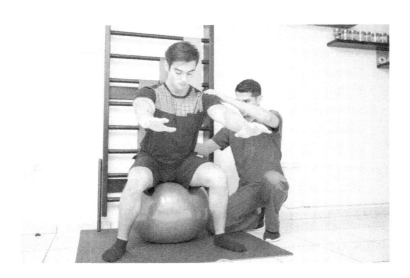

If you've tried conservative chiropractic care or PT and have had no relief or you notice your problem worsening, it's time to see the medical doctor, and in this case, an orthopedic surgeon or pain management specialist. Depending on the source of your back pain, pain management options may be given along with surgical options, if the structural source of pain is at risk of imminently worsening or is preventing you from working or performing tasks of daily living.

I'm sometimes asked about acupuncture or massage as methods of back pain relief. I've had patients try acupuncture with no results and I've had a few patients note relief after treatment. While acupuncture has a long history within eastern medicine, its method of pain relief isn't always going to be effective where cases of severe structural damage are occurring. Also, there are times when a massage will do more harm than good. Whenever you've developed sudden pain due to an injury or even some unknown cause, the inflammation period time clock starts ticking and takes about 48-72 hours to wind down. During this time, you'll want to stick to only using ice therapy as mentioned earlier in this chapter.

Getting a massage while you're in the inflammation period will tend to stir up tissues that are already damaged and will aggravate any swelling already taking place. Massage performed during the wrong time has a similar effect as using heat therapy at the wrong time; it feels great while it's happening, but you feel like you were hit by a truck the next day.

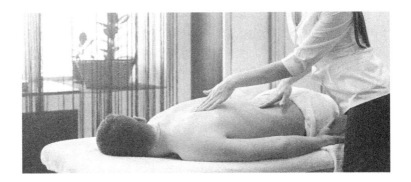

The best time to get a massage for neck or back pain is when the inflammation period has passed, which is generally two to three days after the onset of pain. By this point, the inflammation and swelling has gone down and tissue repair is taking place. Massage therapy done during this period will help ensure the muscle fibers heal in the proper direction and minimize the chances of scar tissue forming.

1234567891011121314̠15

[1] Jensen M, Brant-Zawadzki M, Obuchowski N, et al. Magnetic Resonance Imaging of the Lumbar Spine in People Without Back Pain. N Engl J Med 1994; 331: 69-116.

[2] Hoy D, March L, Brooks P, et al The global burden of low back pain: estimates from the Global Burden of Disease 2010 study Annals of the Rheumatic Diseases Published Online First: 24 March 2014. doi: 10.1136/annrheumdis-2013-204428

[3] Vallfors B. Acute, Subacute and Chronic Low Back Pain: Clinical Symptoms, Absenteeism and Working Environment. Scan J Rehab Med Suppl1985; 11: 1-98.

[4] The Hidden Impact of Musculoskeletal Disorders on Americans, United State Bone and Joint Initiative, 2018.

[5] Rubin Dl. Epidemiology and Risk Factors for Spine Pain. Neurol Clin. 2007; May;25(2):353-71.

[6] Sauver, JL et al. Why patients visit their doctors: Assessing the most prevalent conditions in a defined American population. Mayo Clinic Proceedings, Volume 88, Issue 1, 56 – 67.

[7] Hartvigsen J et al. Low Back Pain Series: What Low Back Pain Is and Why We Need to Pay Attention. Lancet, June 2018; Volume 391, Issue 10137; p2356-2367.

[8] In Project Briefs: Back Pain Patient Outcomes Assessment Team (BOAT). In MEDTEP Update, Vol. 1 Issue 1, Agency for Health Care Policy and Research, Rockville, MD.

[9] Katz JN. Lumbar disc disorders and low-back pain: socioeconomic factors and consequences [review]. J Bone Joint Surg Am. 2006;88(suppl 2): 21-24.

[10] Time to recognize the value of chiropractic care? Science and patient satisfaction surveys cite usefulness of spinal manipulation. Orthopedics Today 2003 Feb; 23(2):14-15.

[11] Bigos S, Bowyer O, Braen G, et al. Acute Low Back Problems in Adults. Clinical Practice Guideline No.14. AHCPR Publication No. 95-0642. Rockville, MD: Agency for Health Care Policy and Research, Public Health Service, U.S. Department of Health and Human Services, December, 1994.

[12] Chou R, Hoyt Huffman LH. Nonpharmacologic therapies for acute and chronic low back pain: a review of the evidence for an American Pain Society/American College of Physicians Clinical Practice Guideline. Ann of Internal Med 2 Oct. 2007;147(7):492-504.

[13] Bronfort G, Haas M, Evans R, et al. Evidence-informed management of chronic low back pain with spinal manipulation and mobilization. Spine. 2008;8(1)213-225.

[14] Goodman D, Burke A, Livingston E. Low Back Pain. JAMA. 2013; 309(16):1738.

[15] Goertz C et al. Effect of Usual Medical Care Plus Chiropractic Care vs. Usual Medical Care Alone on Pain and Disability Among U.S. Service Members With Low Back Pain: A Comparative Effectiveness Clinical Trial. JAMA Network Open.

74

# 17

# When Can You Exercise Again?

When you have a sudden flare-up of back pain, the worst thing you can possibly do is try to exercise yourself back to normalcy. The presence of back pain means you have damaged tissues that aren't able to provide you with normal function. Exercising too much before they are healed will only make the pain last longer and cause complications leading to more back pain episodes down the road.

If you are undergoing back pain treatment currently, your doctor may allow you to start exercising again on a minimal basis simply to get more activity into the tissues to promote healing. As your pain and function improves, your exercise level may be raised gradually to return you to your normal pre-injury or pre- back pain state. Your doctor may recommend changing exercises you've done before or give you new exercises to do to strengthen your back, balance your posture, and make sure the back pain episodes you've had in the past don't come back to haunt you again in the future.

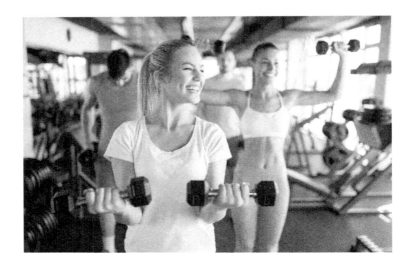

Every back pain situation is different. Knowing when a patient can return to normal exercise is figured out on a case-by-case basis that has as much to do with what the patient is doing when out of the office as it does when they're in the office. Any patient who wants to return to normal exercise activity should follow their doctor's recommendations as closely as possible and try not to do too much too soon. Most people who are avid exercise aficionados are rabid about keeping up with their workouts and always pushing themselves relentlessly. This is a recipe for disaster if the proper amount of time is not taken to reset the tissues and come up with a plan to make sure that future episodes of pain do not occur like before.

# 18

# Do You Need Back Surgery?

As a chiropractor, it's out of my scope to say whether someone should or shouldn't have surgery on their lower back. However I've seen enough cases to know when my chiropractic care is going to have a limited effect and that surgery could be a viable option. When I see those kinds of patients, I try to give them every option from chiropractic to physical therapy to self-care, up to and including referral for a surgical consultation.

Having a surgical consultation is not a death sentence. In some cases, surgery is the only and best option. Those cases typically involve patients that have intractable pain preventing them from doing their daily activities, or nerve problems so severe that there's either muscle atrophy, twitching of the muscles, or loss of feeling so severe that normal daily function is being impaired. In those cases, surgeons will usually try to fix the problem using the most conservative methods available.

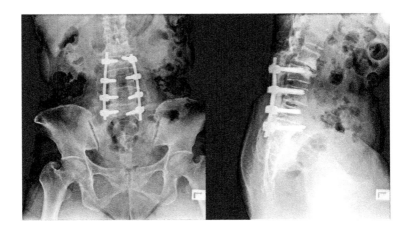

The success and failure rates for lower back surgery are still inordinately high compared to other types of surgery, so it's best to try to avoid it whenever possible. However, if all other conservative options have been exercised and there is no symptomatic change, any patient in this situation should consider a consultation with a surgeon — or possibly more than one — to get different opinions about what can be done.

IMPORTANT NOTE: Just because a patient may need surgery or had surgery done on their back or neck doesn't mean they are no longer a candidate for chiropractic care or massage or physical therapy. That would be like saying you no longer need to brush or floss or see your dentist just because you got a root canal or a crown. It simply means the area that needed surgery now may need to be avoided or treated differently as the other areas of the spine are co-managed. Don't forget; there are 24 bones in the spine. Surgery on one, or two, or three of them might be necessary in some cases, but the other 20+ vertebrae will still need lifelong attention – like your teeth – to make sure *they* won't need surgery down the road.

# 19

# The Most Commonly Overlooked Cause Of Back Pain

Back pain is extremely common. As we already know, it's a condition that most of us will face at some point during our lifetime. And as you've probably seen, there is no shortage of pills, rubs, shots, and treatment devices available to manage back pain.

However, the majority of back pain treatments do nothing to address WHY someone has back pain. These treatments only seek to reduce the symptoms felt by the patient instead of eliminating the source of those symptoms.

Since we are bipedal creatures — meaning, we walk upright on two feet — it's vital we have a level foundation for our spine to rest on. By default, this means our pelvis must be level, which means our legs must be of equal length when standing up barefooted on a level surface. (See figure x.)

Due to the inherent nature of our bodies, we aren't perfectly symmetrical from one side to another. You might notice this on yourself, or when looking at other people, how, perhaps, one ear may look slightly lower than the other, or one eye might be slightly smaller or larger than another. On women, it's not unusual sometimes for one breast to be larger than another or for one to be positioned lower than the other. These variances are extremely common, but most are simply not big enough to be seen with the naked eye.

So what happens when someone has a difference in length on one leg versus the other? The result is an unlevel pelvis when that person is standing or walking. The pelvis will tilt downward on the lower leg side, which causes the lower spine to lean in the same direction. It's common, then, for the rest of the spine to begin to bend back the other direction away from the short leg side in an attempt to find postural balance. This can result in what's known as a postural scoliosis.

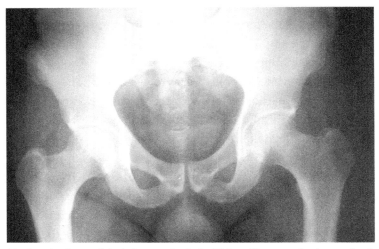

*Notice the lower hip joint on the left. This will cause the lower back and pelvis to tilt, resulting in chronic back pain.*

In a postural scoliosis, there are uneven forces being placed on the muscles, joints and discs. And while the body may be very good at compensating for these forces over the short term, long term imbalanced forces allow the degenerative aging process to be accelerated, causing premature wear and tear responsible for many of the aches and pains patients see us for. In effect, staying in a crooked position for extended periods of time causes your muscles, joints, and discs to age rapidly and become older than the rest of you.

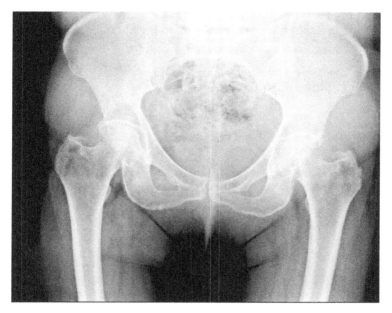

*Notice the right hip and leg lower than the left.*

Knowing this, we must then evaluate leg length inequality in chronic lower back pain cases whenever possible. The average person has a leg length difference of approximately 3 millimeters, while back pain sufferers with leg length inequality will often have a difference of 6 millimeters or more. The most severe case of leg length difference I have seen in practice was an 18 year old female in excellent physical condition except for the lower back pain she suffered from.

After x-ray analysis, it was determined that one of her legs was 36 millimeters shorter than the other. That's about an inch and a half! To know what that felt like, go find one of your shoes that has a sole thickness of about an inch and a half, put it on, but leave the other shoe off. Now walk for five minutes. That crazy, crooked and twisted feeling you'd experience is what her young spine had gotten used to.

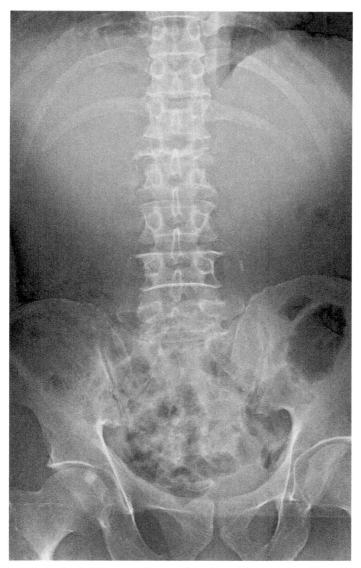

*The leg on the left is seen shorter than the right, causing the pelvis to tilt and creating an unstable foundation for the back to rest upon.*

Whenever leg length inequality is suspected, a standing lumbar x-ray that shows the hip joints is necessary to determine the actual amount of difference. Some health care providers opt for an eyeball measurement of the leg length difference by simply checking visually if one leg is longer than the other while the patient is laying down on a table. Some PTs and even some MDs have been taught to use a tape measure to evaluate the length from the bony point at the front of the hip to the outside edge of the ankle and comparing each side. Both this and the "eyeballing it" method are extremely error prone and not accurate enough to determine a measurement for treatment. Only the standing x-ray, done properly, has enough accuracy to observe the actual amount of leg length difference.

Once the leg length difference has been identified, a rubber heel lift is usually given to the patient to wear in their shoe. This heel lift raises the short leg side up so that it matches the length of the other leg, essentially balancing the pelvis and providing a level base for the spine to rest on. In cases where the leg length difference is 12 millimeters or less, a heel lift is the preferred method of leveling the pelvis. When the leg length difference is more than 12 millimeters, a sole lift on the entire shoe is recommended to correct the first 12 millimeters. The sole lift is preferred over the heel lift alone because lifting the heel more than 12 millimeters causes excessive strain on the ankle joint that can be avoided by lifting the entire shoe.

Once the first 12 millimeters is corrected with a sole lift, any remaining difference can be finished with a heel lift. Of course, the entire amount of leg difference can be corrected with only a sole lift, but many people opt for the smallest sole lift possible so their shoe modification isn't so obvious when they're out in public. Personal preference plus the doctor's recommendation will determine the right course of action.

I call leg length difference the most common overlooked cause of back pain because that's exactly the case. So many health care providers focus on immediate pain relief via spinal manipulation, massage, electrical stimulation, ultrasound, traction, stretching, and exercises. And while these modalities are all excellent when it comes to pain relief, the end result of their use is a flexible, pain free but *imbalanced* spine that, given enough time, will build up enough wear and tear to start the pain cycle all over again or cause a greater risk of injury when performing normal daily tasks. Correcting any structural deficiencies caused by a leg length difference is the best way to ensure that gravity places minimal forces on our backs and we are maximizing the useful life of our discs, muscles, bones and joints.

# 20

# The Pain-Relieving, Arthritis-Fighting, Energy-Regaining, Injury-Preventing, Flexibility and Strength-Building Stretch Sequence

The following simple stretches have been prescribed to my patients for nearly 20 years and are extremely effective in reducing pain, improving flexibility, and reducing injury. By improving flexibility, we increase our range of motion, which helps our joints become more effective at carrying loads placed on them, thus minimizing injury and degeneration as we age.

It is best to do these stretches a minimum of once a day. Feel free to do them more often if you choose. Just make sure you only stretch to the point of resistance and slightly beyond; do not stretch to the point of pain.

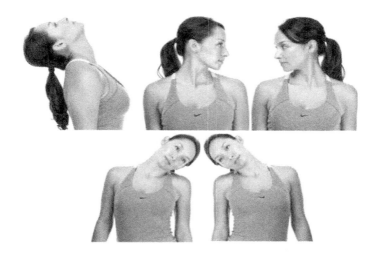

## Head Rotations, Side Bends, and Extensions
### (NO Forward Bending)

Turn your head in each of the directions above for 30 seconds, a minimum of once a day.

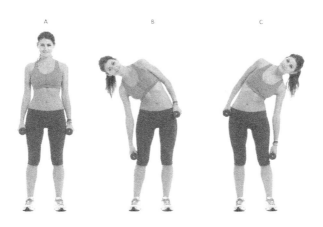

## Spinal Side Bends
(Hold each position for 30 seconds.)

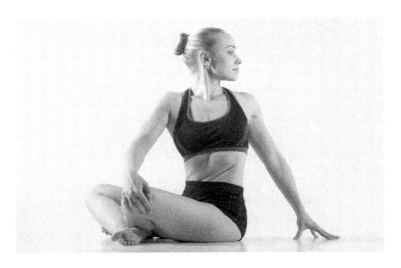

## Spinal Twists
(Hold each side for 30 seconds. These may be done in a chair also.)

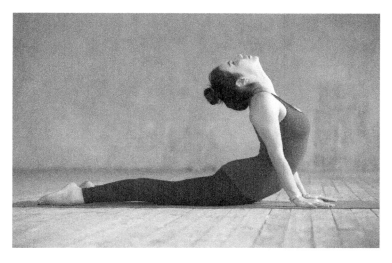

**Spinal Extensions**
(Hold position for 30 seconds.)

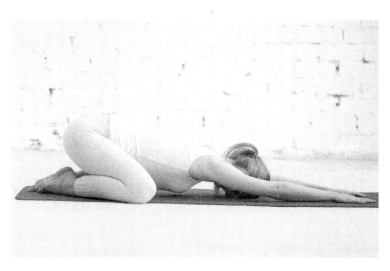

## Child's Pose
(Hold position for 30 seconds.)

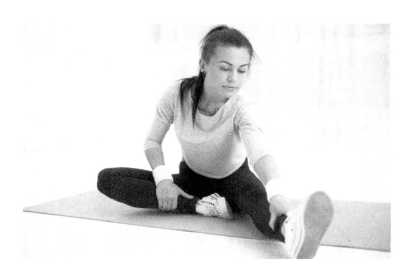

## Hamstring Stretches
Hold 30 seconds each side

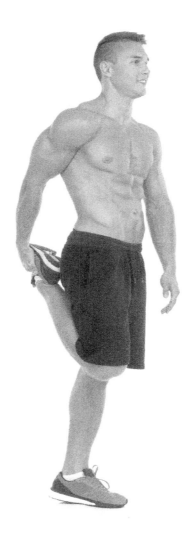

**Quadricep Stretches**

Hold 30 seconds each side

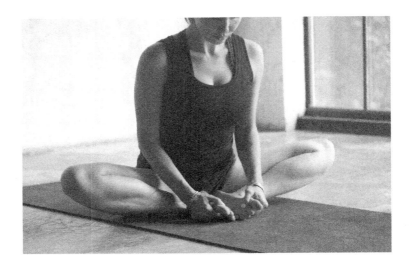

**Butterfly Stretches**

Hold for 30 seconds

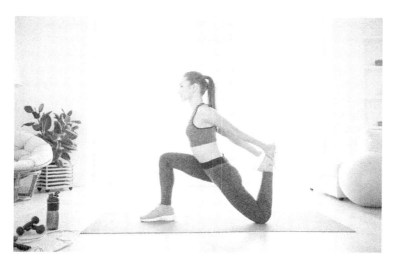

**Hip Flexor Stretches**

Hold 30 seconds each side

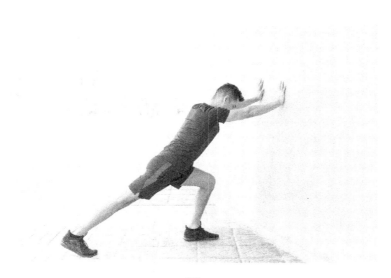

## Calf Stretches

Hold 30 seconds each side

# 21

# Conclusion

If you follow the instructions in this book, you'll have less back pain, more flexibility, and you'll be able to do virtually everything in your life easier. If you have any further questions about your own back pain, you can get in touch with me at jeffkeysar@gmail.com

Thank you for buying this book. It is my sincere wish that the information inside helps you live a more enjoyable, pain-less or pain-free life.

Yours in health,

Dr. Jeff Keysar, DC

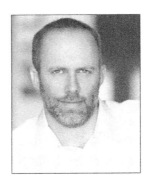

# About the Author

Dr. Jeff Keysar has been a chiropractor for over 20 years and has practiced in Arizona and Nevada. He has treated every type of patient, from babies just days old to seniors 95 years young. His work has helped professional athletes, Las Vegas Strip performers, moms, dads, and children of all ages and conditions.

Correction of acute and chronic back pain is Dr. Keysar's specialty. Through detailed questioning, specific testing, and a focused approach, Dr. Keysar is often able to identify and correct sources of back pain previously overlooked by other health care providers.

*"The key to back pain relief is more than just treatment. It's also finding every contributing lifestyle factor and modifying or eliminating them one-by-one. When you cut off what is feeding your back pain, the pain starves and dies."*

*Dr. Jeff Keysar, D.C.*

Printed in Great Britain
by Amazon

27699398R00059